How to Banish Tendonitis

An Ultimate Guide

to Tendonitis Treatment and Relief

Nathan Wei, MD, FACP, FACR
Director
Arthritis Treatment Center
71 Thomas Johnson Drive
Frederick, Maryland 21702
(301) 694-5800
www.arthritistreatmentcenter.com

DISCLAIMER

This book should not be a substitute for a thorough examination by your physician. The products that are mentioned in this book are recommended. Prior to using any of them, we recommend you seek advice from a qualified specialist. Neither the publisher nor the author may be held liable for any injury, loss, or damage sustained by anyone who relies on the information contained in the book.

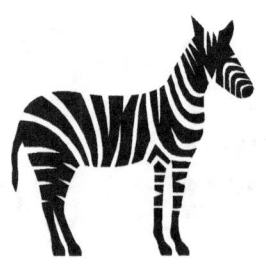

Foreword

Tendonitis is one of the more common disorders seen by physicians, particularly rheumatologists.

These disorders are often chronic and difficult to manage.

The diagnostic and treatment approach to tendonitis has improved dramatically in the last five years.

This book is an attempt to distill the most important aspects of up-to-date diagnosis and treatment... to give the reader an easy to use, relatively comprehensive, one source document to refer to.

I've attempted to create an easy to understand guide; as a result, much of the medical terminology has been defined in layman's terms.

Table of Contents

Chapter One

Introduction

Tendonitis is a set of soft tissue disorders closely related to other problems such as bursitis, ligament strain, and muscle contusions.

Tendonitis is often referred to as a "non-articular disorder." The term "non-articular disorder" refers to pain and limited function occurring in structures that surround and support joints. Because of their location, these conditions are often mistaken for arthritis.

In most studies, soft tissue disorders are the most common problem seen by rheumatologists in practice and occur with a prevalence of about 18 per 1,000 people.

Conditions causing tendon pain are referred to by different names including tendonitis, tendinitis, tendonopathy, and tendinosis... so if you see any of these labels, they all mean the same thing.

Tendons serve as a source of pain generally because of overuse or repetitive injury. When tendonitis exists, there is tenderness and pain that is reproduced by pressure and specific range of motion testing on physical examination.

A number of tendons travel through a fibrous sheath. Inflammation of the lining of this sheath is known as "tenosynovitis." Tenosynovitis may result from trauma, repetitive use injury, systemic inflammatory diseases, or infection. Narrowing and/or inflammation of a tendon sheath may interfere with smooth movement of the tendon.

For example, a "trigger finger" occurs when the flexor tendons of the hand cannot pass smoothly through the fibrous sheaths of the fingers and become caught.

Other conditions where pain and sticking of the tendon (termed "entrapment") occur and are related to tenosynovitis include DeQuervain's tenosynovitis, carpal tunnel syndrome, and tarsal tunnel syndrome. When tendon injury or inflammation becomes chronic, rupture of the tendon may occur.

Causes

Most forms of tendonitis are caused by direct trauma, repetitive use injury, systemic inflammatory diseases, or infection.

Who is affected?

Tendonitis, bursitis, and other overuse syndromes are very common, affecting young, middle-aged, and older adults. Traumatic conditions are more common in young adults. Males are slightly more often affected than females.

Contrary to popular opinion, inflammation is not the underlying problem in tendonitis. Microscopic tissue studies often reveal very few inflammatory cells at the site of pain. This could account for the observation that non-steroidal anti-inflammatory drugs (NSAIDS) often are ineffective in the treatment of this disorder.

It is felt by most authorities that tendonitis is more of a *degenerative* condition.

Confusion with other problems

As mentioned earlier, tendonitis can often be mistaken for arthritis... and vice-versa. Another type of tissue that can become injured and be confused with tendonitis is ligament injury. Ligaments attach one bone to another and provide structural integrity for the skeleton. Injury to ligaments usually results from the application of excessive force. Such "sprains" range in severity from mild partial tears to complete disruption of the ligament with resultant instability of the joint.

The place where ligaments and tendons insert into bone (the enthesis) may also be a site of inflammation. Enthesitis can result from trauma, but may also be associated with systemic inflammatory diseases such as ankylosing spondylitis.

Bursae are small fluid-filled sacs located near joints. They function to cushion the joint from injury and also help tendons and ligaments to glide more easily. Since bursae are located near tendons, bursal inflammation (bursitis) is often either confused with tendonitis or actually may accompany tendonitis.

What does a tendon do?

Tendons have a number of different functions including:
- Stabilization of joints
- Transmission of a load... when a muscle contracts, the tendon has to do the "heavy" lifting
- Protect muscles from damage

What's a tendon made of?

Tendon tissue has a different composition depending on where you look. For example, in the middle of a tendon, you will see mostly Type 1 collagen bundles arranged in a long axis distribution. Tendon cells are called "tenocytes."

Where the tendon inserts into bone is called the enthesis. Here, tendon fibers are more rounded and there is a gradual transition of tendon tissue to cartilage to bone.

Tendon tissue is also structurally different at different areas. For example, at locations where a tendon inserts into muscle, where the tendon slips through soft tissue pulleys that anchor the tendon down, and also where the tendon rubs up against ligaments and bone, tendon tissue is "tougher." This is because at these locations, tendons must resist the stress that comes with shearing forces that act on the tendon.

Different tendons also have different composition depending on where they are located. They also undergo "remodeling" at different rates. For example, highly stressed tendons like the rotator cuff undergo remodeling and repair much more often than tendons where there is less stress.

Tendons have small blood vessels and nerves which help nourish the tendon and provide innervation (the ability to feel).

A tendon has two layers, an inner layer called the endotendon and an outer layer called the epitendon which helps the tendon to heal after injury.

Interestingly, tendon injury undergoes repair when stem cells differentiate into new tendon cells.

(This repair phenomenon is the basis for one of the newer treatments that will be discussed later in this book.)

What tendons are affected the most by tendonitis?

Tendons that are more highly stressed, more often exposed to repetitive strain, and more often associated with more compressive loading or shearing are the ones that develop tendonitis.

Also, the site where tendons will develop tendonitis is usually in areas where there are fewer blood vessels and therefore less of a blood supply.

Examples of tendons that most often are affected by tendonitis include the biceps tendon, the supraspinatus tendon of the rotator cuff, the tendons of the elbow (medial and lateral), the patellar knee tendon, Achilles tendon, and the posterior tibial tendon located along the inside part of the ankle.

A number of changes occur at the cellular level in tendons as they develop tendonitis. For instance, the cells within the tendon become rounder. Also, more blood vessels begin to grow in areas where pain is most extreme.

In the laboratory, elevated levels of destructive enzymes have been shown to be present within tendons that are developing tendonitis.

Clinical findings

Often, a careful history and physical examination can pinpoint the specific cause of the patient's complaint. However, it may sometimes be difficult to differentiate tendonitis from arthritis or other processes. Often tendonitis, bursitis, or enthesitis can be identified as producing "point tenderness" and may cause pain on active motion (when the patient initiates movement), but not passive motion (when the doctor moves the limb).

Different maneuvers during the physical examination may also be helpful for making a diagnosis.

Chapter Two

Shoulder

Biceps tendonitis

This tendon is located on the front of the shoulder. While it has a sheath lined with synovial tissue (the same kind of tissue that lines joints), it is located outside the shoulder joint.

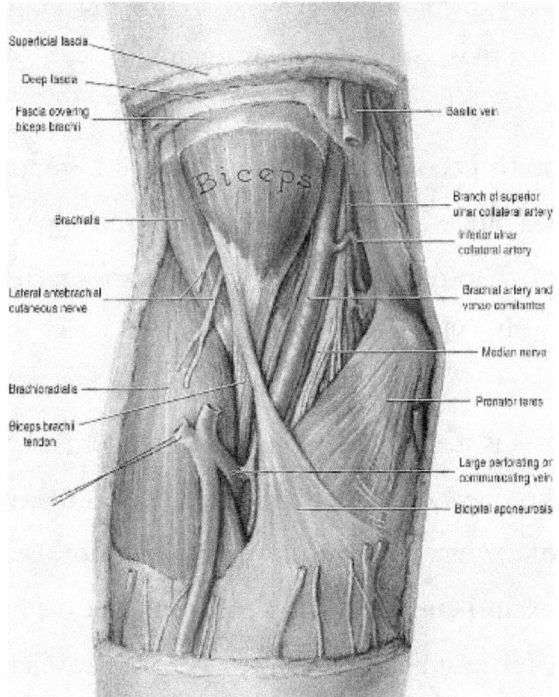

Biceps tendon

Diagnosis

Bicipital tendonitis often presents with pain located at the front of the shoulder. Pain often comes from the long head of the biceps tendon, which runs through a tendon sheath in the bicipital groove of the humerus (upper arm bone) at the shoulder.

Pressure placed on the tendon at the front of the shoulder often generates pain.

The biceps has two parts: the long head and the short head. It is the long head that most often develops tendonitis.

If the tendonitis becomes chronic, it can lead to rupture of the tendon. This causes a bulge in the biceps region of the upper arm. For those of you old enough to remember Popeye, the cartoon character, this is referred to as the "Popeye sign."

The diagnosis is made by demonstrating tenderness of the tendon in the biceps groove. Also, there is a specific test that works because the long head of the biceps is the power supinator of the forearm when the elbow is flexed (bent). What this means is that the biceps is responsible for turning the forearm clockwise when the elbow is bent. (Picture tightening a screw using a screwdriver.) Since this is the case, if the patient complains of pain in the biceps groove area when supination is resisted with the elbow flexed, that is pretty good evidence that biceps tendonitis exists.

Treatment

Treatment begins with accurate diagnosis. Clinical examination and history are usually helpful. The diagnosis can be confirmed using diagnostic ultrasound or magnetic resonance imaging (MRI).

The initial treatment consists of ice, rest, avoidance of high demand overhead activities such as tennis and swimming, and non-steroidal anti-inflammatory drugs (NSAIDS).

Physical therapy modalities such as ultrasound and iontopheresis (driving a small amount of steroid into the region using electrical current) also may be effective.

Many patients will fail these conservative measures and require steroid injection. When injection is performed it should be done with ultrasound guidance to ensure proper placement of the medication; otherwise, the injection will not be as effective and there is also the potential for damage to the tendon and subsequent tendon rupture.

Rarely, removal of the acromion - a part of the shoulder blade that can pinch the biceps tendon - is indicated in people with chronic bicipital tendonitis who remain symptomatic after all conservative measures have failed.

Rotator Cuff Tendonitis

The most common cause of shoulder pain is rotator cuff tendonitis.

This problem is caused most commonly by using the arms for repetitive overhead activities, trauma, arthritis, and calcium deposits.

Background

Four muscles and their tendons make up the rotator cuff of the shoulder. These muscles (the supraspinatus, infraspinatus, subscapularis, and teres minor) start at the scapula (shoulder blade), pass through a tunnel of ligaments on the underside of the collar bone and insert on the humerus (upper arm bone). The tendons merge and form a "cuff" of tissue as they insert on the humerus. (Figure 1)

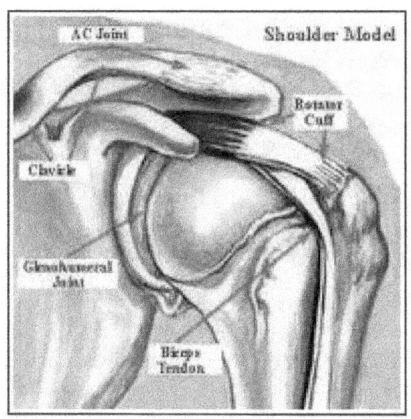

Figure 1
Rotator cuff

They function to lift the arm out, rotate the arm in and rotate the arm out. This allows the upper arm to move freely in all directions. The rotator cuff tendons also form the roof of the shoulder joint. The rotator cuff tendons are separated from the deltoid muscle, which lies on top of the rotator cuff, by a large bursa called the subacromial bursa.

A young rotator cuff is relatively resistant to degeneration. That's why "full thickness" (i.e. complete) rotator cuff tears are unusual in people under the age of 40. When cuff problems develop in younger people they are usually partial thickness or may include complete tearing of the tendon away from bone.

With partial thickness tears, eventual scarring and disuse leads to limited range of motion.

The rotator cuff tendons degenerate with age, which is why rotator cuff problems tend to be more common as people grow older. The blood supply to the rotator cuff is not very good to begin with and as the arm is raised to the side, the rotator cuff becomes pinched between the humerus and the acromion which is the lateral (outside) part of the scapula. This unfortunate anatomic flaw may explain why the rotator cuff is prone to injury in this area.

With increasing age and disuse, less force is required to tear the rotator cuff. Acute symptoms that occur periodically as the cuff becomes more and more torn are usually attributed to "tendonitis." When the acute flare clears up, the shoulder no longer hurts and all that is left is a mild residual weakness. Over time though, a patient can present with a massive rotator cuff tear and minimal symptoms.

Tears of this nature can occur in both shoulders at the same time. It's been estimated that 55 percent of patients will have these bilateral degenerative rotator cuff tears.

Tears of the rotator cuff can progress as major episodes of tearing or by smaller tears that "add up" over time.

A good way of looking at it is to take a piece of paper and grip the top two corners and try to tear it. Now take the same piece of paper and put a small tear at the top in the middle and now pull each corner.

Once these rotator cuff tears start, it is difficult for the tears to heal because, excessive loads are placed on the shoulder mechanism, and the blood supply is not so good.

As each group of rotator cuff fibers is torn, that places more stress on the remaining fibers. Also, as the tear progresses, the muscle that the tendon is attached to pulls more making the defect larger.

Most tears start with the supraspinatus and progress to involve the infraspinatus, teres minor, and then the subscapularis tendons. Also as the tear progresses, it may actually also affect the biceps tendon.

Diagnosis

When the rotator cuff is torn, pain is felt when the muscles are contracted. This pain limits the ability of the rotator cuff muscles to stabilize the shoulder joint.

One of the major functions of the rotator cuff is to resist the pull of the deltoid muscle. The deltoid lifts the head of the humerus up into the shoulder socket while the rotator cuff, when healthy, resists this pull. As the rotator cuff weakens because of chronic tendonitis and tearing, the weakened rotator cuff allows the humeral head to rise under the pull of the deltoid. When the humeral head is pulled upward it squeezes the rotator cuff against the acromion (part of the shoulder blade).

Over time, not only is the rotator cuff damaged more, but there is also damage to the head of the humerus and the glenoid labrum of the scapula (the cup that the humerus interacts with).

This degenerative process is aggravated by chronic overuse (e.g. manual labor involving repetitive shoulder movements against force) or by arthritis in nearby joints. An example would be a person with rheumatoid arthritis who has arthritic involvement of the shoulder joint or the acromioclavicular joint (the joint that joins the shoulder blade to the collar bone).

Rotator cuff problems tend to evolve over time. For instance, initial involvement with mild tendonitis may progress, resulting in a complete tear of the rotator cuff tendons.

Also, mild tendonitis may cause the patient to favor the affected arm, leading to less movement of the affected muscles. This allows the deltoid muscle to pull the humeral head higher in the shoulder socket, which in turn reduces the space through which the rotator cuff tendons must pass. This may result in "impingement" (pinching) of the rotator cuff against the acromion (part of the shoulder blade), which can cause further pain and worsen the entire process.

When this becomes chronic, shortening of the tendons may occur which greatly decreases movement of the shoulder. This "frozen shoulder" syndrome is called adhesive capsulitis.

Those at risk for rotator cuff tendonitis include: elderly people, those with inflammatory arthritis of the shoulder (such as rheumatoid arthritis), diabetics, alcoholics, athletes who engage in repetitive overhead or throwing movements, carpenters, welders, and painters.

In some cases, particularly in younger persons (e.g. baseball pitchers), injury to the rotator cuff is sudden and acute. More commonly, pain related to rotator cuff dysfunction arises slowly and often becomes chronic.

Symptoms

Patients with rotator cuff problems complain of shoulder pain. The pain is usually somewhat difficult for the patient to localize. Often, the patient will say "it's deep and achy."

Many patients complain of waking at night because of the pain. It is often worsened by movements that require specific use of the affected muscles.

However, patients may compensate and perform movements that normally use the rotator cuff muscles by using other muscles to move the arm. For instance, a patient may use his trapezius muscle (the muscle alongside the neck at the top of the shoulder) to lift the shoulder. A patient may use the other arm or the smaller muscles in the lower arm to do chores.

A patient may also avoid using shoulder muscles altogether.

Patients with rotator cuff problems are usually able to lift their arm forward or backward but they have a lot of difficulty lifting their arm out to the side because of pain or because of weakness.

If it is severe, for example, in someone with long standing disease and adhesive capsulitis, passive movements (i.e. done by the physician) may be limited or result in pain.

While all tendons may be affected in the rotator cuff, the most frequently affected tendon is the supraspinatus tendon.

The other rotator cuff muscles and tendons can also be a source of pain and should be assessed.

In some cases, it may be possible to differentiate tendonitis from a complete tendon tear. However, it is often difficult to differentiate between the two.

Complete tear of the rotator cuff usually occurs after trauma. Patients also complain of shoulder pain and weakness and may have a positive "drop arm test." This is a test where the doctor lifts the arm up at the side and asks the patient to hold the arm in place. With a complete rotator cuff tear, the patient will have difficulty holding the arm up.

Symptoms of rotator cuff tendonitis are variable. The problem may present with acute symptoms with intense pain developing within a day. On the other hand, symptoms can smolder, getting better then getting worse over weeks to months. The pain can be present with the arm dangling down but becomes worse when the arm is raised to the side. Even simple activities like combing or brushing hair can be so painful that they are avoided. Aching pain can be present at night and be made worse by sleeping on the affected side. There may be local tenderness at the side of the shoulder or upper arm.

So how does rotator cuff tendonitis present to a doctor? On examination, the various joints around the shoulder are inspected and they are not tender. These joints include the sternoclavicular (the joints that join the breastbone to the collarbone), the acromioclavicular (the joint that joins the collarbone to the shoulder blade), and the glenohumeral joint (the joint where the humerus joins the shoulder blade).

There is pain noted when the deltoid muscle (the thick muscle on the side of the upper arm) is pressed and the patient may have trouble lifting the arm to the side because of pain.

The physician may lift the arm out at the side then externally rotate the shoulder (turn it out so that it looks like you're trying to say "Hi"). This motion may magnify the pain of rotator cuff tendonitis. Lifting the arm out to the side, then internally rotating it (like you're getting ready to scratch your lower back) also can irritate the rotator cuff.

The history and physical examination is usually sufficient to make the diagnosis if the physician being consulted is knowledgeable and experienced.

For confirmation either magnetic resonance imaging or diagnostic ultrasound may be helpful. X-rays are useful for identifying arthritis in the acromioclavicular joint or in the glenohumeral joint. Sometimes x-ray will pick up abnormal calcium deposits.

Magnetic resonance imaging and diagnostic ultrasound can confirm the diagnosis and are mandatory before initiating treatment.

Treatment

Rotator cuff treatment follows a typical algorithm. Non-steroidal anti-inflammatory drugs supplemented by physical therapy, local measures such as ice and heat, as well as topical agents are usually started.

Physical therapists will often prescribe range of motion and strengthening exercises along with therapeutic ultrasound, electrical stimulation, and iontopheresis.

Exercises to do

The following exercises may help you (see pictures 1, 2 and 3). Ask your doctor if you should do other exercises too.

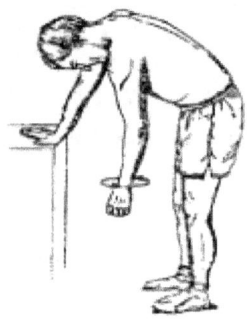

Picture 1

Picture 1. – Range of motion. Stand up and lean over so you're facing the floor. Let your sore arm dangle straight down. Draw circles in the air with your sore arm. Start with small circles, and then draw bigger ones. Repeat these exercises 5 to 10 times during the day. If you have pain, stop. You can try again later.

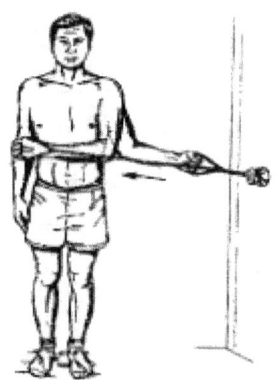

Picture 2

Picture 2. – Rotator cuff strengthening. Use a piece of rubber tubing for these exercises. Stand next to a closed door with a doorknob. Loop the tubing around the knob. With your hand that is closest to the door, bend your arm at a 90° angle and grab the loop of the tubing. Pull the band across your tummy. At first, do 1 set of 10 exercises. Try to increase the number of sets as your shoulder pain lessens. These exercises should be done every day.

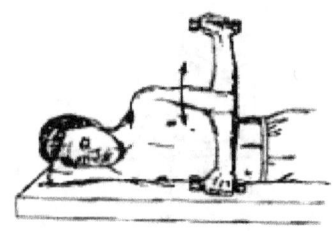

Picture 3

Picture 3. – Upper extremity strengthening. As your pain goes away, try adding a general upper body weight-lifting program using weight machines or free weights. Lie on your right side with your left arm at your side. With a weight in your left hand and your forearm across your tummy, raise your forearm. Keep your elbow near your side.

More recently cold laser (low level laser) has been used with some degree of success by some practitioners.

In many cases, particularly when the tendonitis is chronic, steroid injection may be called for. Again, ultrasound guidance is mandatory to ensure proper placement of the medication.

In patients who do not respond to steroid injection, percutaneous tenotomy and autologous tissue grafting using platelet-rich plasma (PRP) is an excellent option.

Chronic, degenerative rotator cuff tears should probably not be operated on. This differs from the management of acute tears in young athletes where arthroscopic surgical techniques are generally well tolerated and usually effective.

Calcific tendonitis

Calcific tendonitis is a common form of tendonitis of the rotator cuff. Calcium deposits form, usually in the supraspinatus tendon, about 1-2cm from the insertion of the tendon into the humerus (upper arm bone). Fifty percent of patients with calcific tendonitis have shoulder pain with acute and chronic restricted range of motion.

Twenty to thirty percent of patients have both shoulders involved. The cause of this specific condition is unknown but could be related to insufficient blood flow, chronic degeneration of the tendon, or metabolic problems.

Diagnosis

Symptoms are similar to that for rotator cuff tendonitis. Sometimes, severe pain may be experienced at night.

Treatment

The treatment for this condition has been less than satisfactory. Surgery usually works but there is a high risk of operative complications.

Arthroscopic procedures fail about half the time.

Shock wave therapy has been used to disintegrate the calcium deposits. Uncontrolled studies have demonstrated that the deposits are partially or completely obliterated in two-thirds of patients and symptomatic improvement occurs in 75 percent of patients.

A needle aspiration procedure done using local anesthetic relieves symptoms in up to 75 percent of cases and relieves symptoms in more than half the patients. Diagnostic ultrasound guidance is required for this procedure to be optimal.

Of the non-invasive techniques, only therapeutic ultrasound has been shown to be effective. In one study involving 63 patients, half of whom were assigned to ultrasound treatment and the other half to sham (placebo), 42 percent of the ultrasound treated group improved at 9 months compared with only 8 percent of the sham group. (Ebenbichler GE, et al. New Eng J Med 1999; 340:1533-8). It was noted by the authors that some patients in other studies report a short term increase in symptoms at the beginning of ultrasound treatment.

Another advantage of ultrasound is that it is relatively inexpensive.

The mechanism by which ultrasound works is unknown.

One other type of treatment - non-steroidal anti-inflammatory drugs (NSAIDS) - may be useful for symptoms in some patients. NSAID treatment needs to be monitored closely because of the potential development of side effects.

Recently, the use of ultrasound guidance with needling of the calcific deposit as well as tenotomy (poking small holes in the affected tendon) and autologous tissue grafting using platelet-rich plasma seems to work very well.

Adhesive capsulitis

Also termed "frozen shoulder," this condition is characterized by pain and loss of shoulder motion in all four planes. The cause may be unknown or it may occur in the face of diabetes, thyroid disease, a pinched nerve in the neck, or malignancies involving the lung.

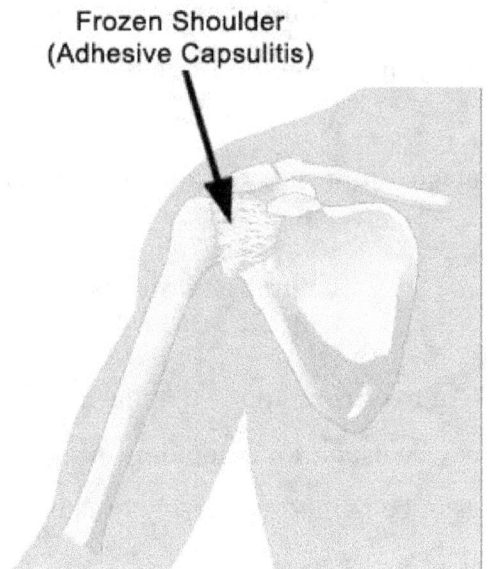

Frozen Shoulder
(Adhesive Capsulitis)

Frozen shoulder

Night time pain is common.

The diagnosis is suspected on clinical grounds, confirmed by the exam, and supported by the results of magnetic resonance imaging studies.

Treatment consists of non-steroidal anti-inflammatory drugs, physical therapy with stretching of the cuff, and injection of glucocorticoids using ultrasound needle guidance.

More recently, percutaneous needle tenotomy with autologous tissue grafting (platelet-rich plasma) has been successful.

Rarely, arthroscopic surgery with debridement or manual decompression of the shoulder under general anesthesia is required. The latter approach can cause arm fracture as a complication and should be reserved for the most difficult of cases.

Chapter Three

Elbow

There are three major types of tendonitis that occur at the elbow: lateral epicondylitis (tennis elbow); medial epicondylitis (golfer's elbow); and triceps tendonitis.

Lateral epicondylitis

By far, the most common tendonitis in this area is lateral epicondylitis. Pathologically, what occurs are microscopic tears and incomplete repair of the common tendon of the extensor muscles of the forearm as it inserts on the lateral epicondyle of the humerus (upper arm bone). This is the outside part of the elbow. If you lay your arm down flat on a table with the top of the hand facing the ceiling, the lateral epicondyle is the part of the elbow that also faces the ceiling.

Lateral epicondylitis often results from overuse (e.g. repetitive rotation of the forearm muscles such as using a screwdriver or a hammer) or extending the forearm against resistance for extended periods of time (hitting a one-handed backhand in tennis). Another way that lateral epicondylitis starts is by trauma - accidentally hitting the outside part of the elbow against a doorframe, for example.

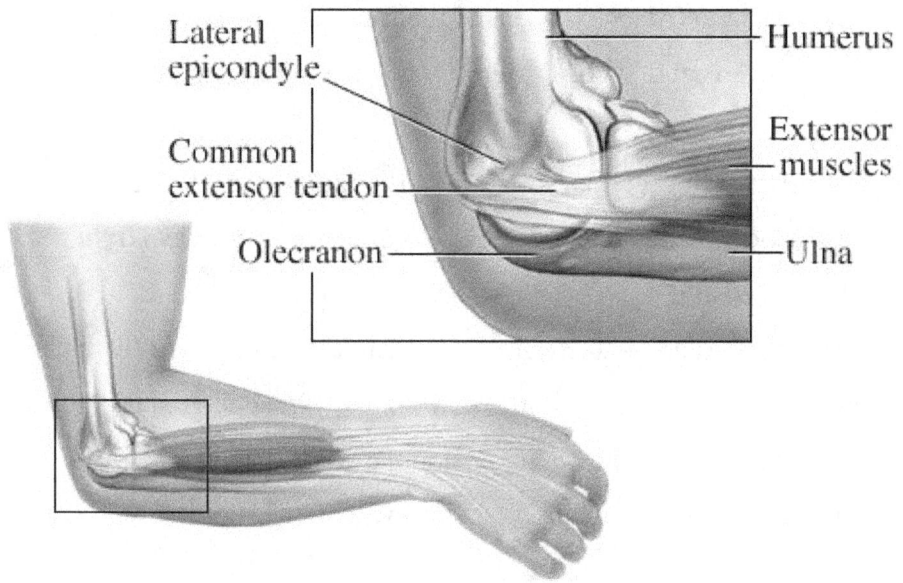

Lateral epicondyle

Diagnosis

Patients complain of pain at the lateral epicondyle during work or during recreation. Physical examination often reveals tenderness over the lateral epicondyle and pain with resisted extension of the wrist. Pain can be so severe that simple tasks such as getting milk out of the refrigerator or even shaking hands can be excruciating.

The diagnosis is primarily a clinical one. However, there are pitfalls. A nerve, called the posterior interosseous nerve which runs near the lateral epicondyle can become entrapped and look like lateral epicondylitis. Also 5 percent of the time patients have both lateral epicondylitis and posterior interosseous nerve entrapment.

Entrapment of other nerves such as the radial sensory nerve and musculocutaneous nerve can also look like lateral epicondylitis.

Another "fooler" is tendonitis involving the insertion of the biceps tendon. The biceps tendon has two ends. One end is in the shoulder. The other end attaches to the inside part of the radius (one of the two forearm bones) just beyond the elbow.

Finally, various types of arthritis conditions can cause elbow pain that may be confused with lateral epicondylitis.

The point is: don't automatically assume that a patient with lateral elbow pain has lateral epicondylitis without examining them carefully!

Diagnostic ultrasound and magnetic resonance imaging can help add more diagnostic proof to the clinical impression. Sometimes electrical studies like electromyography and nerve conduction testing can help with the diagnosis of nerve entrapment.

Treatment

Treatment for this condition is both varied as well as controversial. Early in the course, non-steroidal anti-inflammatory drugs and splinting may help. The type of splint used is one that prevents extension of the wrist. Also, a circumferential forearm band that has self-adherent surfaces (i.e. Velcro™) worn just below the elbow can relieve symptoms. The band restricts the motion of the finger and wrist extensor muscles. This relieves the stress on the tendons at the lateral epicondyle.

Physical therapy modalities such as ultrasound, electrical stimulation, iontophoresis, and phonopheresis have produced mixed results. Stretching and strengthening exercises can be beneficial.

Steroid injections are sometimes effective for relieving pain and inflammation. Unfortunately, there are problems associated with this procedure including thinning of the skin at the site of injection, and depigmentation at the site of injection. No more than three injections should be administered. Ultrasound guidance is mandatory.

Surgery has been advocated for lateral epicondylitis that has not responded to conservative measures. Various procedures including release of a contracted capsule, debridement, and so on have their advocates. Prognosis following surgery is dependent on the correctness of diagnosis, skill of the surgeon, possible secondary gain (i.e. a patient stands to gain if they don't get better), and lack of complications.

Newer therapies though seem to have relegated the role of surgery to a back seat position. In patients who fail to respond to other conservative measures, percutaneous tenotomy with autologous tissue grafting with platelet-rich plasma (PRP) using ultrasound guidance has provided excellent results.

Medial epicondylitis

Sometimes referred to as golfer's elbow, medial epicondylitis is less common than lateral epicondylitis. Sometimes seen in golfers, it is also seen in people with manual labor occupations such as bricklayers. It is due to stress at the site of the insertion of the forearm flexor tendons at the medial epicondyle (inside part of the elbow).

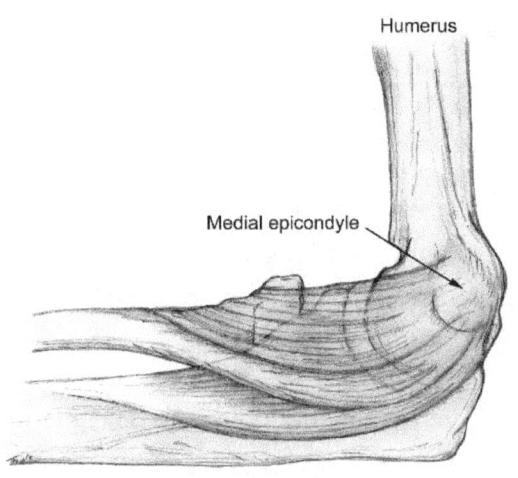

Medial (inside) view of the right elbow

Medial epicondyle

Pain over the insertion of the common flexor tendon at the medial epicondyle is the key to diagnosis. In addition to these conditions, other causes of elbow pain include inflammatory arthritis of the elbow joint and ulnar nerve entrapment (with tenderness on palpation of the ulnar nerve groove at the back of the elbow and signs of ulnar nerve problems... often consisting of numbness and weakness of the fourth and fifth fingers) should be excluded.

Compression of the ulnar nerve can be present in up to 30 percent of people with medial epicondylitis.

The cause of this condition is usually stress on the flexor/pronator muscles (the muscles that bend the wrist down and turn the wrist counterclockwise). This can cause irritation of the flexor muscle origin at the medial epicondyle - the inside part of the elbow.

This can be an occupational and recreational hazard in that people who scale fish or skin animals, along with golfers, tennis players, and baseball players are often affected.

It is very important to exclude ulnar nerve problems.

The diagnosis of medial epicondylitis can be confirmed using either diagnostic ultrasound or magnetic resonance imaging. Electrical testing such as electromyography and nerve conduction testing can help exclude ulnar nerve entrapment.

Treatment

Conservative management includes non-steroidal anti-inflammatory drugs, rest, splinting and physical therapy. Steroid injection is sometimes helpful. Surgical results are mixed.

This is another situation where tenotomy and autologous tissue grafting with platelet-rich plasma (PRP) can be effective.

Triceps tendonitis

The triceps tendon connects the rear of the elbow joint to the triceps muscle. Triceps tendonitis causes pain in the back part of the upper arm near the point of the elbow.

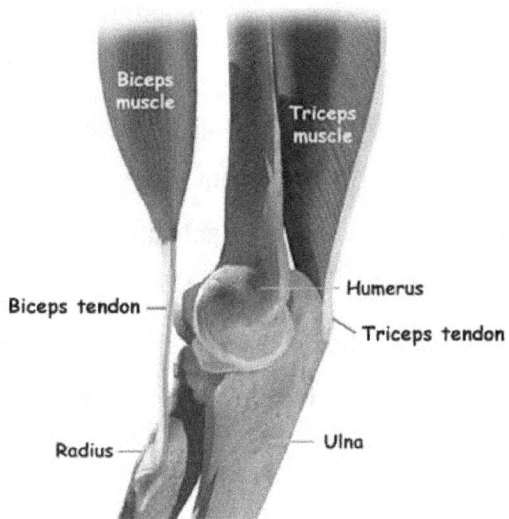

Triceps tendon

Triceps tendonitis occurs from overusing the upper arm and may occur with activities such as throwing and hammering. It may also be caused by a direct blow to the triceps muscle or tendon.

Symptoms can include pain when straightening the elbow or fully bending the elbow. There may be tenderness at the triceps muscle and tendon as well as swelling of the triceps insertion at the elbow.

The diagnosis can be made by clinical examination. To support the diagnosis, either diagnostic ultrasound or magnetic resonance imaging can be used.

Treatment consists of local measures such as ice, non-steroidal anti-inflammatory drugs, supportive strap, and physical therapy.

The best way to prevent triceps tendonitis is to avoid overuse of the upper arm and elbow. It is important to recognize early symptoms so the injury is not worsened by over activity.

Percutaneous needle tenotomy with autologous tissue grafting using platelet-rich plasma (PRP) is an excellent treatment option.

Chapter Four

Wrist and Hand

One of the primary causes of hand and wrist disability is tendonitis. A number of problems may arise in this area. There are two sets of tendons: the flexors on the palm side of the wrist and the extensors on the dorsal (top) of the hand. The tendons reside within a sheath of synovium... the same tissue that lines joints. The synovium provides a cushioned, lubricated surface for the tendons to glide in. Small slips of tissue serve to anchor the tendon sheaths firmly.

The functional anatomy of the hand and wrist tendons is complicated and will not be dealt with here.

When inflammation occurs in the tendon sheath of the hand or wrist, because synovium is involved along with the tendon, and the tendon sheath is an enclosed space, the signs, symptoms, and causes differ from tendonitis that occurs in other large joint areas.

For example, there are multiple causes of tendon inflammation besides overuse. These include infection, diabetes, hypothyroidism (low thyroid), rheumatoid arthritis, lupus, gout, and pregnancy.

Discussion of these various causes is beyond the scope of this book.

The most common form of tendonitis seen in the wrist is probably related to over-activity. The treatment is straightforward: rest, ice, splinting, non-steroidal anti-inflammatory drugs, and physical therapy.

If there is an underlying condition such as rheumatoid arthritis responsible for the problem, then more aggressive management of that problem is indicated.

Diagnosis

Tendonitis in the wrist may be difficult in some cases to distinguish from other problems such as arthritis and carpal tunnel syndrome. In addition, these latter two problems may coexist with tendonitis in the wrist.

Trigger finger

Tendonitis in the fingers often presents with locking and clicking. While the trigger may be subtle such as a simple give in the finger, it may be more pronounced with permanent locking of the finger in the flexed position. In other words, the finger can be bent but not straightened without taking the finger and manually straightening it.

Attempts to bend the finger result in a catching sensation. This condition is referred to as "trigger finger." The cause of trigger finger is swelling of the synovium inside the sheath leading to inability of the tendon to glide smoothly and getting caught by one of the slips of tissue (called "pulleys") that anchor the tendon sheath.

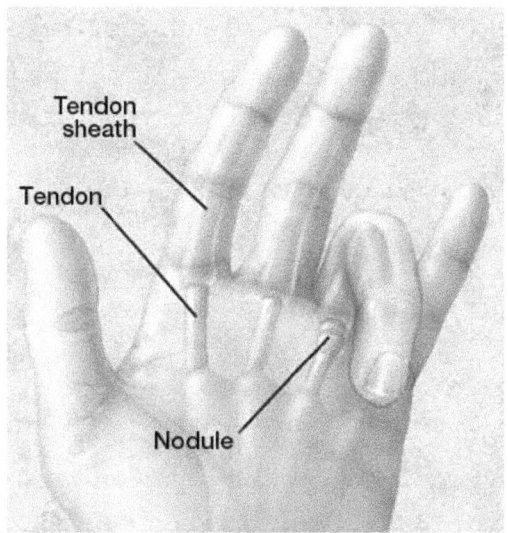

Trigger finger

The diagnosis of trigger finger is made clinically. Diagnostic ultrasound will often locate the exact spot where the tendon is being trapped.

Treatment early consists of the use of splinting and non-steroidal anti-inflammatory drugs. Judicious use of steroid injections with ultrasound needle guidance by an experienced physician will often be curative. (Anderson B, et al. Arch Int Med 1991; 151: 153-6)

In cases where glucocorticoid injections do not work, an injection of large volumes of fluid, along with cutting the pulleys, using a small needle with ultrasound guidance has been reported to be successful.

In rare instances, surgery may be required.

DeQuervain's tenosynovitis

A unique type of tendonitis may occur along the radial side of the wrist. This is termed DeQuervain's tenosynovitis. This is a painful condition that affects the abductor pollicis longus and the extensor pollicis brevis tendons of the thumb.

De Quervain's Tenosynovitis

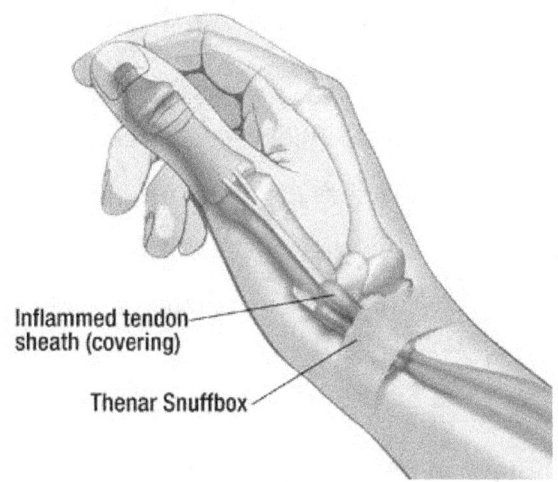

Inflammed tendon
sheath (covering)

Thenar Snuffbox

DeQuervain's tenosynovitis

DeQuervain's tenosynovitis is more common in women than men.

It is often associated with recent pregnancy or repetitive use of the thumb and wrist.

Patients may drop objects from their hands or be unable to lift a baby or change diapers without experiencing excruciating pain.

Diagnostic confusion may arise if the patient also has osteoarthritis at the base of the thumb or carpal tunnel syndrome. Both of these conditions may also occur along with DeQuervain's disease.

Clinical examination shows localized swelling and tenderness along the outside of the thumb extending into the wrist.

Pain is felt along the radial (thumb) side of the wrist and is aggravated by bending the thumb across the palm, placing the fingers over the thumb, then pushing the wrist to the ulnar side (little finger side) at the same time. This is called Finkelstein's maneuver.

The treatment involves the use of non-steroidal anti-inflammatory drugs, splinting that immobilizes the thumb during activities that aggravate the pain, and corticosteroid injection using ultrasound needle guidance.

Occasionally, tenotomy with instillation of platelet-rich plasma (PRP) may work well for chronic conditions.

If a patient fails these treatments, surgery is indicated.

Acute flexor tenosynovitis

Some patients can experience an acute infection of the tendon sheath in the hand. The cause is a bacterial infection due to staph or strep. Frequently, small abrasions, puncture wounds, and penetration of foreign bodies may precede the development of this condition.

The patient presents with severe pain, tenderness, and swelling of the finger. Spread of the infection into the rest of the hand and wrist can occur if not treated immediately. Hand surgery consultation is the immediate treatment approach of choice. The patient will require drainage, debridement, and biopsy.

On occasion, the above condition can be due to calcium deposits rather than bacteria. It is a difficult distinction to make. A hand surgeon should still be consulted to be on the safe side.

Single sheath tendonitis of the finger

Some patients can present with a single swollen finger. This may be due to a foreign body, tumor (giant cell or pigmented villonodular synovitis), tuberculosis, sarcoidosis, calcium deposits, fungus, crystals (gout, pseudogout), or malignancy of the lining of the tendon sheath (sarcoma).

While steroid injection may be useful, a patient with this type of presentation should be worked up for a number of associated diseases. Surgical exploration is almost mandatory to make sure that malignancy or indolent infection is not present.

Proliferative tendonitis

Tendonitis involving several fingers at one time can occur in the face of conditions such as rheumatoid arthritis, systemic lupus erythematosus, scleroderma, and psoriatic arthritis. The treatment consists of local measures but also implies that the patient needs tighter control of their systemic illness.

Depuytren's contractures

Depuytren's contracture is a fibrous thickening of the soft tissue in the palm of the hand. It tends to affect middle-aged men and older people primarily of Northern European descent.

It is associated with conditions such as tobacco smoking, trauma, diabetes, manual labor, alcohol abuse, and the long term use anti-seizure drugs.

It is usually bilateral - meaning it affects both hands. There is thickening of the soft tissue of the palm with the formation of tender fibrotic cords. As the disease progresses, there is gradual drawing in of the fingers with inability to fully straighten the fingers out. The ring and little fingers are affected most often.

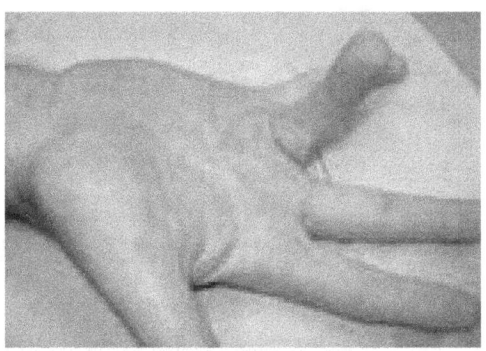

Depuytren's contracture

The condition has been seen in association with trigger fingers, carpal tunnel syndrome, lateral epicondylitis, and frozen shoulder.

Progression of this condition is unpredictable but the course tends to be progressive.

Various treatments have been tried with mixed success.

The treatment of choice until recently was surgical release. Results with this procedure have been determined by the duration and severity of the condition.

More recently, other less drastic types of treatment have been introduced.

One treatment is a minimally invasive procedure referred to as needle aponeurectomy. In this procedure, the abnormal tissue is weakened using a small needle in the palm.

Another treatment involves the use of a device that treats the condition using pulsed sound waves (Health Sonix).

Xiaflex is a drug (Auxilium Pharmaceuticals) which consists of a material called collagenase which breaks down the connective tissue that forms the Depuytren's contracture. It is injected directly into the contracture. It is FDA approved.

Chapter Five

Hip

Tendonitis occurs in the hips generally as a result of overuse. The typical patient is a young (or not so young) person who is very active and who participates in activities such as cycling, running, or sports such as football and soccer.

The hip joint is a ball and socket. The femoral head (top of the upper leg bone) is shaped like a ball and articulates (interacts) with the acetabulum (socket) of the pelvis.

The hip joint is subjected to strong forces during weight-bearing activities due to the long, lever-arm mechanism of the leg, with the hip joint being the fulcrum. That is one major reason why osteoarthritis affects the hip so often.

Strong ligaments and muscles provide stability of the joint with movement.

In the front of the hip there are multiple muscles such as the rectus femoris, iliopsoas, gracilis, and sartorius muscles that connect the pelvis to the femur.

They are responsible for flexing the hip (bringing the knee up towards the chest).

These muscles, along with the rest of the quadriceps muscles, which straighten the knee, are the largest and most powerful muscles in the body.

Along the inside of the thigh are muscles that connect the inner part of the femur to the front of the pelvis. These muscles bring the leg back to the middle.

On the outside part of the leg are muscles that move the leg away from the midline. In the back of the leg are other muscles that extend the leg back from the body.

Many muscles also aid in rotating the hip both in and out.

Tendons in the hip are subject to high tensile strength, meaning they must stretch as the muscles shorten.

Tendons are often cushioned from the underlying bone by a lubricating and cushioning sac called a bursa. The largest bursa in the hip joint is located between the iliopsoas muscle in the groin and the pelvic brim and is called the iliopsoas bursa.

The greater trochanter of the femur is a portion of bone that sticks out from the side of the proximal femur.

Trochanteric bursitis

The trochanteric bursa is located here. The trochanteric bursa lies beneath the muscle and is the largest synovial bursa in humans. Pain from the bursa or adjacent tendons of the tensor fascia latae (the thick wide piece of tendon at the side of the hip) and lateral quadriceps muscles is usually caused by an overuse injury, trauma, or inflammatory arthritis.

Trochanteric Bursitis

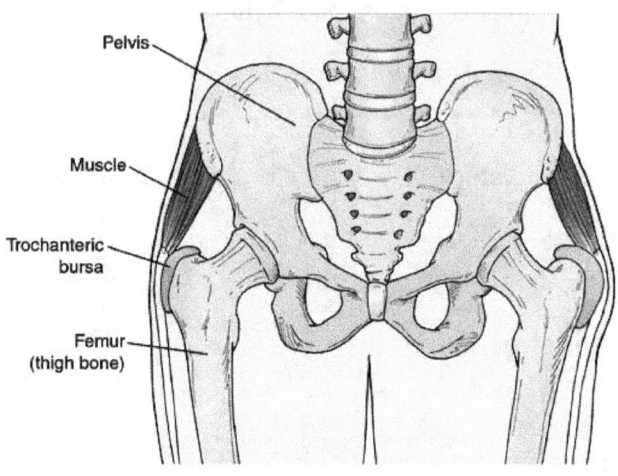

Chronic pain at the front of the hip in the groin may result from iliopsoas or rectus femoris tendonitis.

A snap may be felt with bending and extending the hip. This condition can come on as a result of activities such as running and jumping.

The patient will complain of groin pain that is worsened with extension or flexion of the hip. Getting out of a car or walking up steps can aggravate the pain.

Gluteus medius syndrome

Gluteus medius syndrome is a type of tendonitis that can start after a sudden fall, prolonged weight bearing on one leg for long periods, overuse, or athletic injuries. This condition is most common in middle-aged women who start a vigorous work out program too eagerly and too intensely.

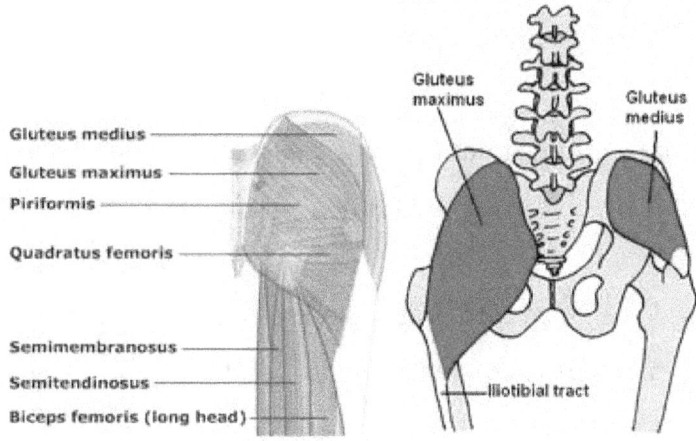

Gluteus medius syndrome

They can present with pain, limp, and weakness. These symptoms can be aggravated by a leg length difference.

Exercises that focus on lifting the leg out to the side, at least at the beginning - should be avoided because they make the tendonitis worse.

As the acute pain resolves, strengthening of the hip abductors will be important. Doing this in the pool may be useful for avoiding re-injury.

It is often difficult to tell the difference between trochanteric bursitis and gluteus medius tendonitis because they are located so close to each other.

Bringing the hip towards the midline is performed by adductor muscles. They originate on the pubic bone and insert onto the upper part of the inner femur.

Adductor or groin strains are commonly seen in athletes involved in sports that involve sudden stopping, starting, and cutting.

Increased risk of adductor strains occur in those with decreased adductor strength, poor conditioning, insufficient stretching, and a history of previous strains.

The hamstrings function as hip extensors. These muscles originate from the ischial tuberosity of the pelvic bone and attach onto the medial tibia and lateral fibula (the two lower leg bones).

Acute hamstring injuries occur with the sudden acceleration movements. Risk factors for these problems are insufficient warm-up, poor flexibility, or decreased strength from previous hamstring strains. Acute hamstring injuries most often occur within the mid belly of the muscle, but rupture where the muscle and tendon meet also can occur.

Treatment

The treatment of trochanteric bursitis involves the use of thermal modalities (ice initially, then moist heat), non-steroidal anti-inflammatory drugs, gentle stretching, and physical therapy. Injection of corticosteroid into the affected bursa can also be helpful. This should be done using ultrasound needle guidance.

Injections into the iliopsoas bursa for bursitis in this area also can be performed by experienced clinicians using ultrasound guidance.

More recently, treatment using ultrasound guided percutaneous needle tenotomy (poking holes in the tendon with a needle) has shown to be beneficial. The theory is that this procedure restarts the healing process by increasing inflammation and blood flow into an area. Addition of stem cells and/or platelet-rich plasma seems to hasten healing by causing the laying down of healthy collagen. Patients who undergo these treatments should not use anti-inflammatory medications because these drugs will prevent the inflammation that is critical to the start of healing.

Iliotibial band tendonitis

Snapping hip syndrome is a condition where there is a snap or pop when the hip is flexed and extended. There are a number of causes for snapping hip syndrome. It is usually due to tendons catching on bone when the hip is moved.

The iliotibial band is a thick, wide tendon that lies on the side of the hip joint. The most common cause of snapping hip syndrome is when the iliotibial band snaps over the greater trochanter (the bony outcropping located at the side of the hip joint). If this is the cause of snapping hip syndrome, patients may also develop bursitis in this area as well.

The iliopsoas tendon is the major hip flexor muscle, and the tendon of this muscle runs just in front of the hip joint. This tendon can catch on a bony part of the pelvis and cause a snap when the hip is flexed.

A magnetic resonance scan can be ordered to better define the cause of the snapping hip and to make sure there is not a tear of the hip cartilage which can also cause snapping.

Treatment involves the use of topical agents, thermal modalities, non-steroidal anti-inflammatory drugs and injections of glucocorticoids.

Physical therapy can help by stretching out the muscles and tendons that cause a snapping hip.

Use of ultrasound guided tenotomy with autologous tissue grafting material (platelet-rich plasma) has been reported to be successful.

Surgery is rarely necessary.

Chapter Six

Knee

The two major types of knee tendonitis that can occur are quadriceps tendonitis and patellar tendonitis.

Quadriceps tendonitis

The patella (kneecap) glides up and down inside a groove in the femur (thigh bone) during flexion (bending) and extension (straightening) of the knee. The strong quadriceps muscles on the front of the thigh attach to the top of the patella via the quadriceps tendon. This tendon inserts into the patella, covers the patella, and continues down to form the patellar tendon. The patellar tendon in turn, attaches to the front of the tibia (shin bone). The quadriceps muscles, straightens the knee by contracting (tightening up) and pulling at the patella via the quadriceps tendon. Quadriceps tendonitis occurs when inflammation affects the quadriceps tendon.

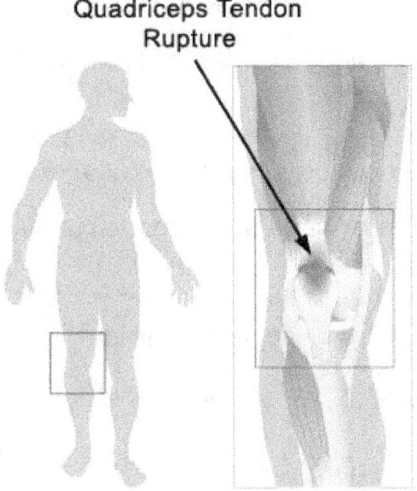

Quadriceps Tendon
Rupture

Quadriceps tendon

Quadriceps tendonitis occurs as a result of excessive stress on the quadriceps tendon. It is seen most commonly in runners and other athletes involved in activities such as quick starts and quick stops. Injury occurs due to overuse leading to microscopic tears in the quadriceps tendon. Pain and inflammation result. Chronic inflammation can lead to rupture.

Quadriceps tendonitis is common in people involved in activities that include a lot of running, jumping, stopping and starting.

Pain is felt just above the patella. There may be swelling and tenderness involving the quadriceps tendon. The pain can vary from being relatively mild to being painful to the point that involvement in any kind of athletic activity is out of the question.

The diagnosis can be suspected by clinical examination and confirmed using diagnostic ultrasound or magnetic resonance imaging.

Treatment includes rest, ice, non-steroidal anti-inflammatory drugs as well as stretching and strengthening exercises.

Percutanous needle tenotomy with autologous tissue grafting using platelet-rich plasma has been reported to be very effective.

Quadriceps tendon problems can be avoided by gradual introduction of jumping or running and by the use of proper training techniques. Off-season strength training of the legs, particularly the quadriceps muscles, can also help.

Patellar tendonitis

Patellar tendonitis is most common in individuals involved in sports where there is frequent jumping — for instance, basketball, soccer and volleyball players. For this reason, patellar tendonitis is commonly known as "jumper's knee."

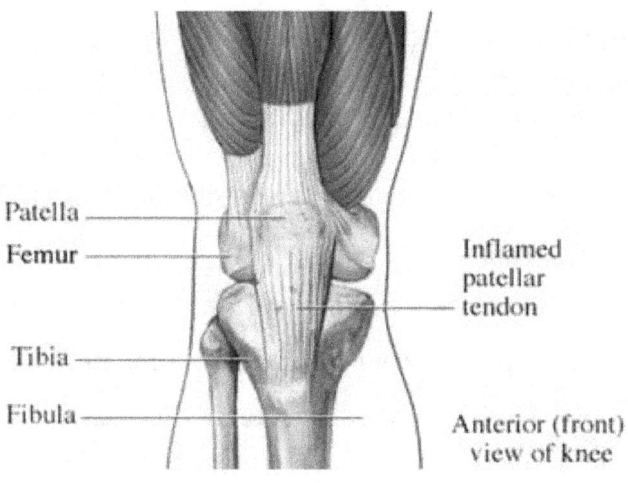

Patella

Femur

Inflamed patellar tendon

Tibia

Fibula

Anterior (front) view of knee

Patellar tendonitis

Diagnosis

Pain is the primary symptom of patellar tendonitis and is located in the region between the patella (kneecap) and tibia (shin bone). The pain may be most acute during physical activity — especially with running or jumping. After a workout or practice, the pain may persist as a dull ache.

The pain may be present at the start of physical activity or immediately after an intense workout. It can then increase in intensity as the intensity of the activity increases. If untreated, it may become continuous. Activities such as going up and down stairs may become very uncomfortable. Nighttime pain may also be a prominent symptom.

Patellar tendonitis is termed an "overuse injury" because it occurs as a result of repeated stress on the patellar tendon. The stress leads to tiny tears in the tendon. As the tears in the tendon become more numerous, the body's attempts to keep up with the healing process are overwhelmed and inflammation becomes chronic.

A combination of factors usually leads to the development of patellar tendonitis.

Excessive intensity and frequency of physical activity, particularly repetitive jumping, is often associated with patellar tendonitis. Sudden increases in the intensity of physical activity or increases in frequency of activity put added stress on the tendon.

Obesity increases the stress on the patellar tendon and increases the risk of patellar tendonitis.

Tight muscles - both the quadriceps group in front and the hamstrings in back - increase the stress on the patellar tendon. A corollary to this is if the muscles are imbalanced with one group being much stronger than another, then this situation also puts excessive strain on the tendon.

The diagnosis is usually made by history and physical examination.

Pain due to patellar tendonitis is located in the front of the knee just below the patella. The diagnosis can be confirmed by using diagnostic ultrasound or magnetic resonance imaging. These studies are also useful for excluding other causes of knee pain that can mimic patellar tendonitis such as tearing of the menisci (cartilage cushions inside the knee) or patellofemoral arthritis which is arthritis occurring in the joint between the kneecap and the femur.

Patellar tendonitis treatment is a long process, no matter what type of treatment you've chosen. Recovery may take a few weeks or months if the injury is not too severe, or as long as a year or more for people who undergo surgery.

Most people with patellar tendonitis find pain relief and improvement using conservative treatment — meaning treatments other than surgery. If you have persistent signs and symptoms for six months or more, you may want to discuss the potential benefits and risks of patellar tendon surgery with your doctor.

Treatment

Treatment is usually conservative to start. Rest is important. This does not mean giving up all physical activity, but a patient should avoid running and jumping. A physical therapist can help establish whether there are improper body mechanics involved that might be aggravating the issue.

Stretching can help loosen inflexible muscles, especially inflexible thigh muscles (quadriceps), which contribute to the strain on your patellar tendon.

Specific exercises to strengthen the patellar tendon and the quadriceps muscles are important.

Eccentric strengthening programs have been shown in some studies to help treat and prevent patellar tendonitis. A strap that applies pressure to your patellar tendon can help to distribute force away from the tendon itself and direct it through the strap instead. This may help relieve pain.

Non-steroidal anti-inflammatory drugs may be useful for symptom relief. Corticosteroid injection is generally not recommended because of the danger of tendon rupture.

Other types of therapy where positive results have been reported include therapeutic ultrasound, cold laser, extracorporeal shock wave therapy, and electrical stimulation.

Resolution of symptoms usually takes weeks to months.

Percutanous needle tenotomy with autologous tissue grafting using platelet-rich plasma has been reported to be very effective.

Surgery is reserved for patients who fail conservative treatment. The recovery time after surgery can be anywhere from six to twelve months.

Iliotibial Band Syndrome

The iliotibial band is a wide, flat structure that originates at the iliac crest – the lateral part of the pelvis. It courses along the lateral upper hip then travels along the side of the thigh and inserts at the lateral aspect of the proximal tibia (outer lower leg bone).

This iliotibial band (ITB) acts as a ligament between the lateral femoral condyle (outside upper leg bone) and the lateral tibia to stabilize the knee. The ITB is responsible for the following motions. It lifts the leg out to the side, helps the hip to rotate internally (turn leg in), and also helps with extension and flexion (straightening and bending) the knee.

ITB syndrome occurs as a result of the ITB rubbing against the lateral femoral condyle. There may also be inflammation of a bursa located near the tibial insertion of the ITB.

Iliotibial band (ITB) syndrome (ITBS) is the most common cause of lateral knee pain among athletes. ITBS develops as a result of inflammation of the bursa surrounding the ITB as well as the tendon next to the bursa. This condition usually affects athletes who are involved in sports that require continuous running or repetitive knee flexion and extension.

Pain along with clicking as the knee is bent and straightened are common symptoms.

Typically, the patient with ITBS presents with the gradual onset of lateral knee pain that is present during running.

Pain is localized over the lateral femoral epicondyle.

If not treated, the pain may eventually radiate to the calf and up the lateral thigh.

Pain is commonly experienced with climbing stairs or running downhill.

Pain at rest is usually associated with severe tendonitis. Other problems that may cause lateral knee pain include a tear in the lateral meniscus.

Physical findings in patients with ITB syndrome include an abnormal gait which is done to avoid the motion of the ITB rubbing against the lateral femoral condyle as well as point tenderness at the lateral femoral condyle and at the tibial insertion.

The predisposing factors include improper warm-up and stretching, increasing the quality and quantity of training sessions too quickly, misalignment of the leg, and worn out or improper athletic shoes.

Treatment

Treatment is aimed at controlling inflammation, correcting poor training habits, and making modifications for anatomic structural variants.

Non-steroidal anti-inflammatory drugs (NSAIDS) can be used to control pain and inflammation.

Any training habits that contribute to ITB syndrome should be avoided.

Corticosteroid injection and physical therapy also can be helpful. Surgery is rarely indicated. Percutaneous needle tenotomy with platelet-rich plasma (PRP) can be helpful.

Popliteus tenosynovitis or tendonitis is a tear in the popliteus tendon. The popliteus tendon connects from the bottom back of the thighbone across the back of the knee to the top front of the shin bone. The popliteus tendon prevents the lower leg from twisting outward when running.

Popliteus tendonitis is often caused when the feet roll inward. Running downhill can also tear the popliteus tendon by putting too much stress on the tendon.

With popliteus tendonitis, inflammation (pain, swelling, and tenderness) is felt on the outside of the knee. With time, scar tissue may form. This may make it painful to exercise and it may take weeks to fully recover from this form of tendonitis.

The most important part of treating this condition is resting the popliteus tendon while it heals. Resting the leg reduces swelling and keeps the tendonitis from getting worse. When the pain decreases, a patient may begin normal, slow movements.

Ice causes blood vessels to constrict which helps lessen inflammation (swelling, pain, and redness). Putting crushed ice in a plastic bag and covering it with a towel and then putting this under the knee for 15 to 20 minutes every hour may help.

A physician may wrap the knee with tape or an elastic bandage to keep the knee from swelling. A patient may be told to keep the leg raised on a stool or pillows which also helps to lessen swelling.

A patient may use ibuprofen and acetaminophen for the pain.

A patient may be referred to physical therapy. A physical therapist will do treatments to help the tendonitis heal faster. Exercises to make the tendon stronger will be started after the tendonitis has healed.

A physical therapist may use ultrasound to increase blood flow to the injured area.

Therapists may use massage to stretch the tissue and bring heat to the injury which increases blood flow. This can help the leg heal faster and better.

A patient may gradually increase the amount of weight they put on the leg when the therapist gives them permission. The patient will be told to make sure they are pain free as they use the leg more.

Shoe inserts with a reinforced heel counter are also useful. This will give better heel control to keep the heel from rolling inward.

A patient should not return to running until they are pain free and the physician says it is OK. He or she should start exercising slowly with activities such as bicycling and running when told it is OK.

A patient should always do stretching exercises first. This will loosen the muscles, especially the hamstring muscle in the back of the thigh. Stretching also helps lessen stress on the popliteus tendon.

A patient should not run downhill for at least 3 weeks after they have started running again once the physician says it is OK.

Chapter Seven

Ankle

There are three major types of tendonitis that may occur at the ankle. On the lateral (outside) part of the ankle are the peroneal tendons. On the medial (inside) part of the ankle run the extensor hallucis and posterior tibial tendons, and in the rear of the ankle is the large Achilles tendon.

Peroneal tendonitis

There are two peroneal tendons. The peroneus longus tendon originates from the top one-third of the fibula (outside lower leg bone), while the brevis originates from the lower two thirds of the fibula. The two tendons run just behind and below the lateral malleolus (the bump on the outside part of the ankle bone). They run through a specific groove and insert into the lateral part of the foot.

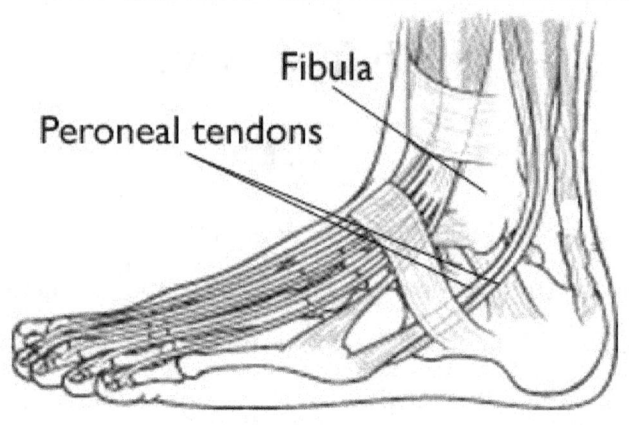

Peroneal tendonitis

Diagnosis

The hallmark of peroneal tendonitis is lateral ankle or foot pain. Over time, loss of the ability to turn the foot out occurs.

In addition to tendonitis, lengthwise tears of the tendon are a common problem.

Subluxation (dislocation of the tendons outside of the groove) of both peroneal tendons may occur following an acute traumatic episode or may be of a more chronic nature.

Symptoms of peroneal tendonitis include pain behind and beyond the lateral malleolus (the bony bump located on the outside part of the ankle). Swelling and tenderness may also be present.

In contrast to that, the symptoms of peroneal tendon subluxation consist of snapping along the outside of the ankle along with a sense of weakness or pain.

Pain with toe walking or cutting laterally while playing on a field also is seen.

With acute injury, pain and swelling are noted over the back and outside of the ankle.

Chronic injuries such as turning the ankle can lead to subluxation which leads to lateral ankle instability and painful snapping across the ankle.

Peroneal tendon tears are the last major concern. With acute injury, pain and swelling are just behind and below the lateral malleolus. The patient may have had pain prior to injury, but now the pain can be debilitating and ankle strength is decreased.

Chronic injury results in constant pain behind the lateral malleolus. This progressively worsens in terms of both function and the level of pain.

Diagnosis is suspected clinically by history and physical examination. Confirmatory evidence can be obtained with diagnostic ultrasound and magnetic resonance imaging.

Treatment

Acutely, most ankle injuries are managed with rest, ice, compression, and elevation (RICE) with or without a short period of no or limited weight bearing. Non-steroidal anti-inflammatory drugs (NSAIDS) can also be prescribed to reduce inflammation and pain. Once the swelling and pain has subsided, a more extensive examination can be performed. If the symptoms are minimal and if no significant instability is present, a rehabilitation program can be started. This program should include an ankle strengthening, flexibility and proprioception (ability of the patient to "feel" the ground) regimen.

In cases of peroneal tendonitis in which the tendon is degenerated but not ruptured, acute care may include 2-6 weeks of cast immobilization, particularly if the symptoms are recurrent.

Conservative treatment is considered a failure if symptoms such as pain and instability of gait continue.

Surgery is rarely if ever indicated for peroneal tendonitis but may be needed for subluxation and tears.

Injection with corticosteroids is controversial since the peroneal tendons are superficial and are located near the sural nerve. Injecting in this area can cause complications such as nerve damage. As a result, only skilled practitioners using ultrasound needle guidance should inject this area. A technique called hydrodissection using ultrasound needle guidance may be particularly useful since this focuses on the tendon sheath and avoids the tendon completely. Following this type of injection, a patient needs to wear an air splint for at least three days following the injection.

As a patient improves, attempts to restore ankle strength, flexibility, and return the patient to their activity should be undertaken. Proprioceptive training is crucial because recurrent sprains are related to poor muscle firing and balance. Every sprain can stretch and damage the peroneal tendon fibers, loosen the outside ankle support, and create further instability.

Chronic tears of the peroneal tendons with persistent pain and instability require surgical repair. Tendonitis may cause nodules or scar tissue that may need surgery.

Good pre- and post-exercise, ankle stretching and continued use of strengthening techniques will help speed recovery.

Posterior tibial tendonitis

The posterior tibial muscle originates at the upper third of the tibia. The tendon takes a course that passes behind the medial malleolus (the bony area that sticks out from the inside of the ankle). The muscle inserts into a number of bones along the inside of the middle of the foot.

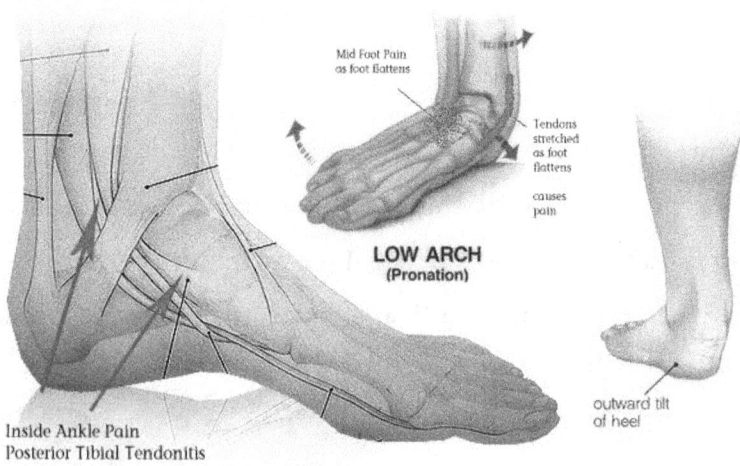

Posterior tibial tendonitis

The posterior tibial tendon helps hold the arch up and provides support for stepping off on the toes when walking. If this tendon becomes inflamed, over-stretched or torn, pain is felt on the inner part of the ankle and the patient begins to lose the inner arch on the bottom of the foot, leading to flatfoot.

Symptoms include pain and swelling on the inside of the ankle, loss of the arch and the development of a flatfoot, pain on the outer side of the ankle or foot, weakness and an inability to stand on the toes, and tenderness over the middle part of the foot, especially during activity.

Posterior tibial tendon dysfunction often occurs in women over the age of 50 years. Several other risk factors may be present. These include: obesity, diabetes, hypertension, previous surgery or trauma, such as an ankle fracture on the inner side of the foot, local steroid injections, and inflammatory diseases such as Reiter's syndrome, rheumatoid arthritis, spondylosing arthropathy and psoriasis.

Athletes who participate in sports such as basketball, tennis, soccer or hockey may tear the posterior tibial tendon. The tendon may also become inflamed if excess force is placed on the foot, such as when running on a banked track or road.

The diagnosis is based on both a history and a physical examination. Clinical examination may demonstrate that the hind-foot—the rear of the foot—is turning out.

Magnetic resonance imaging and diagnostic ultrasound may be used to confirm the diagnosis.

Treatment

Without treatment, the flatfoot that develops from posterior tibial tendon dysfunction will become rigid. Arthritis develops in the hind-foot. Pain increases and spreads to the outside of the ankle. The way a patient walks may be affected and wearing shoes may be difficult.

In the early stages, posterior tibial tendon dysfunction can be treated with rest, non-steroidal anti-inflammatory drugs, and immobilization of the foot for 6 to 8 weeks with a rigid below-knee cast or boot to prevent overuse. After the cast is removed, shoe inserts such as a heel wedge or arch support may be helpful. If the condition is advanced, a custom made ankle-foot orthosis or support may be needed.

Steroid injection along with immobilization is controversial but can be effective if the injection is done with ultrasound needle guidance and the practitioner is skilled. A technique called hydrodissection, using ultrasound needle guidance is particularly useful since it focuses on the tendon sheath and completely avoids the tendon itself.

After such an injection, the patient should be placed in an air-type splint for at least three days following the injection.

With both peroneal tendonitis as well as posterior tibial tendonopathy, percutanous needle tenotomy with autologous tissue grafting using platelet-rich plasma has been reported to be very effective.

If conservative treatments don't work, the physician may recommend surgery. Several procedures can be used to treat posterior tibial tendon dysfunction; often more than one procedure is performed at the same time.

Flexor Hallucis Longus tendonitis

The flexor hallucis longus (FHL) tendon is one of three structures that lie in the tarsal tunnel.

Running behind the medial malleolus (inside ankle bone), the FHL is the most posterolateral (to the rear and side). The FHL runs forward into the foot to insert onto the distal phalanx (the end bone) of the great toe. The FHL acts as a flexor of the great toe, elevates the arch, and assists with plantar flexion of the ankle (pointing the toes away from the body).

Patients with FHL tenosynovitis usually present with pain in the posteromedial aspect of the ankle (behind the inside ankle bone). The pain improves with rest and increases in sports requiring push off and extended running.

Usually no tenderness with pressure is present due to the deep location of the tendon. Pain and weakness are noted with resistance to plantar flexion of the first toe joint (pointing the toe down towards the floor). Pain also may be present in the tarsal tunnel (the area just back of the inside ankle bone).

FHL tenosynovitis typically is associated with repeated push off maneuvers, such as those executed by ballet dancers or sprinters. Sometimes blunt trauma and repetitive impact may also play a role.

FHL tendonitis may occur at three sites. These are: the entrance of the fibro-osseous tunnel between the medial and lateral talar tubercles (the prominent ankle bones on the inside and the outside part of the ankle); the flexor sheath behind the medial malleolus (inside ankle bone); between the sesamoids (small bones) of the great toe.

Among the conditions that can look like this are: Achilles tendonitis, tibialis posterior tendonitis, and tarsal tunnel syndrome.

Clinical findings include: swelling, pain, and tenderness posterior to the medial malleolus; triggering and pain along the tendon sheath that may occur with toe flexion (bending the toe down); and reduced ability to point the great toe up.

Plain x-rays of the foot are helpful with the differential diagnosis and diagnostic ultrasound imaging or magnetic resonance imaging (MRI) can help rule out a tear.

Treatment consists of immobilization, activity restrictions, and non-steroidal anti-inflammatory drugs. Steroid injection is possible but caution must be exhibited because of the nerves and blood vessels in the area.

Surgery is sometimes required.

Achilles tendonitis

Achilles tendonitis is a condition where irritation and inflammation of the tendon in the back of the ankle occurs. Achilles tendonitis is a common overuse injury that often occurs in middle-age recreational athletes. Overuse causes inflammation that leads to pain and swelling. Achilles tendonitis can lead to small tears within the tendon, and make it susceptible to rupture.

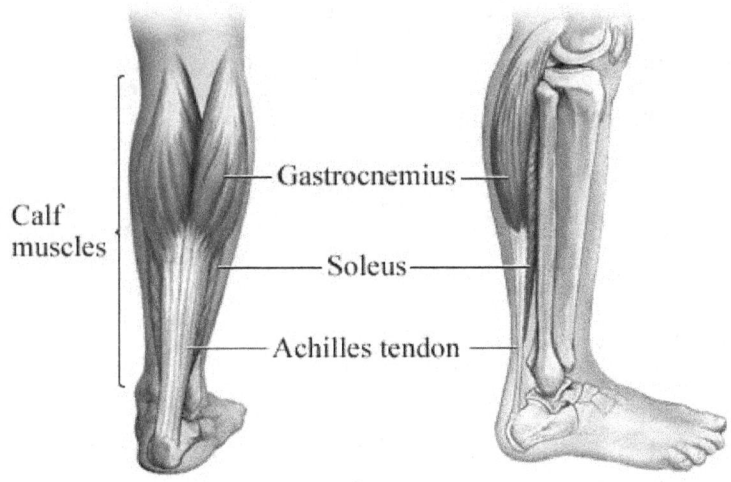

Achilles tendonitis

The two most common causes of Achilles tendonitis are lack of flexibility and overpronation—when the foot rolls inward during walking or running. Other factors associated with Achilles tendonitis are recent changes in footwear and changes in exercise training schedules. Often long distance runners will have symptoms of Achilles tendonitis after increasing their mileage or increasing the amount of hill training they are doing.

Tendons, with increasing age, become less flexible, more rigid, and more susceptible to injury. That is why middle-aged recreational athletes are most susceptible to Achilles tendonitis.

The Achilles tendon may become painful from a number of causes, including direct trauma, improper footwear, repetitive overuse (e.g. with athletic activity), and systemic inflammatory diseases such as ankylosing spondylitis, Reiter's syndrome, and psoriatic arthritis.

The main symptom with Achilles tendonitis is pain at the back of the heel. This is where the tendon inserts on the heel bone. Patients with Achilles tendonitis usually experience the most significant pain after periods of inactivity. As a result, patients tend to experience pain after first walking in the morning and when getting up after sitting for long periods of time. Patients will also experience pain while participating in activities, such as when running or jumping. Achilles tendonitis pain associated with exercise is most significant when pushing off or jumping.

The diagnosis of Achilles tendonitis is suspected by taking a careful history and physical examination.

Pain on pressure is often noted at the bony insertion of the tendon. As the problem becomes chronic, the tendon can become "bumpy" with irregular swelling and have crepitus (crunchiness) with motion. There are also bursae superficial to and deep to the Achilles tendon that can become inflamed and be a source of pain.

Diagnostic ultrasound or magnetic resonance imaging may be helpful in confirming the diagnosis.

Treatment

The treatment starts with recognition of the problem. Rest, non-steroidal anti-inflammatory drugs, and physical therapy may be helpful in the early stages. Having the patient wear shoes with a slight heel may also work. Flat shoes should be avoided.

A retrospective study of 83 athletes with Achilles tendonitis seen from 1976 to 1988 was conducted. (Read MTF, Motto SG. Jour Ortho Med 1993; 15: 74-9.) Patients received local steroid injection into the peritendon region – not into the tendon. The researchers found no increased risk of tendon rupture. Local steroids did not help athletes to return to competition sooner; however, they did help reduce symptoms more quickly. Athletes who were treated earlier did better than athletes who had chronic problems.

Tendonitis and tendon rupture are unusual and unexpected side effects of drugs. Fluoroquinolone antibiotics have been associated with Achilles tendonitis and Achilles rupture.

The treatment of choice now appears to be percutaneous needle tenotomy with autologous tissue grafting. This procedure involves the use of a small needle that is used to puncture the tendon multiple times. Since local anesthetic is used, the procedure is not usually painful. This stimulates the tendon to bleed. Platelet-rich plasma which contains multiple growth factors is obtained from the patient. This material is then injected into the site of injury and tendon healing is stimulated.

Surgery is not indicated unless severe tearing is present.

Chapter Eight

Foot

The foot, because it bears a lot of weight, must have a complicated system of muscles and nerves to aid in weight bearing and proprioception (ability to feel things in space).

As a result, many muscles and tendons are required for proper functioning of the foot.

Plantar fasciitis

One of the most common tendon problems is plantar fasciitis.

The plantar fascia is a cord of tissue that connects the bottom of the heel with the ball of the foot. The function of the plantar fascia is to provide support for the arch of the foot and to assist with shock absorption during foot strike (i.e. walking or running). For instance, during running, the vertical forces in the foot, at foot strike, may reach 2-3 times an individual's body weight. The plantar fascia and arch are also part of the foot's shock absorption system. As a result, the plantar fascia can be a source of substantial pain.

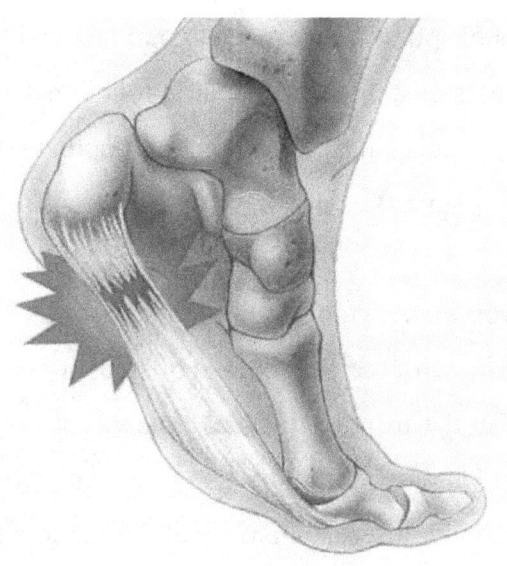

Plantar fascia

Plantar fasciitis is often associated with trauma in the form of excessive activity - for instance, a runner that suddenly increases his or her mileage. Or it may be associated with abnormal foot mechanics or excessive weight. This condition is also associated with a type of arthritis condition called spondyloarthropathies.

Plantar fasciitis is the pain caused by inflammation of the insertion of the plantar fascia on the medial (inner) process of the calcaneal tuberosity (heel bone). Plantar fasciitis may cause significant heel pain, resulting in alteration of a person's activities. This condition sometimes is called "heel spurs."

This term is wrong because many people who do not have symptoms have bony heel spurs, whereas many patients with plantar fasciitis have no bony heel spur. A heel spur is found in 15-25 percent of asymptomatic individuals in the general population; however, many patients with plantar fasciitis have no heel spur on x-ray.

The most prominent symptom of plantar fasciitis is a history of intense sharp heel pain with the first couple of steps in the morning. Pain is experienced at the front of the heel bone, but it may radiate into the ankle. An athlete may complain of a dull ache in the heel at the end of the day, especially after extensive walking or standing.

During activity, the pain usually decreases as the athlete warms up, but it generally returns after activity. The pain is aggravated particularly by sprinting. In more severe cases, the athlete complains of heel pain after periods of prolonged sitting.

Associated symptoms include stiffness in the foot and localized swelling in the heel.

On examination, a doctor may note that pressure over the inner part of the heel can reproduce the pain of plantar fasciitis. In more severe cases, pain may also be reproduced by pressure applied to the bottom part of the heel. Other maneuvers that may reproduce the pain of plantar fasciitis include pushing the toes of the foot up towards the head, which is sometimes called a "windlass" test, or having the athlete stand on the tiptoes and walk.

So what can lead to plantar fasciitis?

Training errors are among the major causes of plantar fasciitis in athletes. Athletes usually have a history of an increase in distance, intensity, or duration of activity that precedes the development of plantar fasciitis.

The addition of speed workouts and hill workouts are particularly high risk behaviors for the development of plantar fasciitis.

Running indoors on poorly cushioned surfaces or with poorly cushioned shoes is also a risk factor.

It cannot be stressed enough that any person starting a vigorous exercise program needs to wear an appropriate shoe type for their foot type.

Athletic shoes rapidly lose cushioning properties. Change them often. One good test: if you bend the sole of the shoe and it bends easily, it's time to change.

Structural risk factors include flat feet, overpronation (meaning the foot at the time of foot strike on the ground turns in too much), high arches, leg length abnormality, and excessive turning of the leg bones during running.

Athletes with low or high arches have increased stress placed on the plantar fascia with foot strike.

Pronation is a normal motion during walking and running, providing foot-to-ground surface contact and impact absorption by allowing the foot to completely absorb the impact. Overpronation, on the other hand, can lead to increased tension on the plantar fascia.

Leg length abnormalities and abnormal leg mechanics can lead to an alteration of running biomechanics, which may increase plantar fascia stress.

Tightness in the calf muscles and the Achilles tendon is considered a risk factor for plantar fasciitis. Reduced ability to turn the toes up has been shown to be an important risk factor for this condition.

Weakness of the calf and foot muscles is also considered a risk factor for plantar fasciitis.

Aging and heel fat pad atrophy are two degenerative risk factors for plantar fasciitis.

There are other possible conditions to rule out before settling on plantar fasciitis as the cause of heel pain. These include entrapment of the posterior tibial nerve (also known as tarsal tunnel syndrome, which is like carpal tunnel syndrome, but in the foot), stress fracture of the heel, bruising of the heel, infection, rupture of the plantar fascia, inflammatory forms of arthritis that can affect the heel, tendonitis due to another cause, and malignancy.

Usually, laboratory studies are not needed in the workup of plantar fasciitis.

X-rays are not helpful for diagnosis. However, diagnostic ultrasound and magnetic resonance imaging can help with diagnosis.

Bony tumor or fracture can occur so a plain x-ray should always be considered in any patient with heel pain, particularly before considering administering a corticosteroid injection.

Magnetic resonance imaging (MRI) or diagnostic ultrasound may be needed to confirm plantar fasciitis or partial and complete plantar fascia rupture.

Bone scans are useful to evaluate for stress fractures, tumors, and infection.

Electromyographic (EMG) studies are useful to evaluate for possible neurologic entrapment syndromes.

Treatment

Initially, patients with plantar fasciitis will be treated with a combination of non-steroidal anti-inflammatory drugs (NSAIDS), stretching exercises, orthotics (arch supports), heel cups, and physical therapy. Physical therapy programs for plantar fasciitis emphasize stretching of the calf and foot. The stretching program should include wall stretches, with the knee in both the extended and flexed positions.

To perform a wall stretch, the patient should stand 3 feet from a wall, placing the hands on the wall. Keeping the toes pointed straight and the heel on the ground, the patient leans the hips toward the wall, and then holds this position for 30-40 seconds. Stretches targeted at the plantar fascia are particularly important.

Ice is best at the start of treatment. Icing should be performed after completing exercise, stretching, and strengthening, and this treatment can be applied by ice massage, ice bath, or ice pack.

For ice massage, the patient can freeze water in a small paper or polystyrene cup and then rub the ice over the painful heel, using a circular motion and moderate pressure for 5-10 minutes.

For an ice bath, a shallow pad is filled with water and ice. The patient soaks the heel for 10-15 minutes. To prevent cold injuries, the patient should use neoprene toe covers or keep the toes out of the ice water.

An ice pack can be made by placing crushed ice in a plastic bag that is wrapped in a towel. The use of crushed ice allows the ice pack to be molded to the foot and increases the contact area; a good alternative is a bag of prepackaged frozen peas or corn wrapped in a towel. Ice packs are usually placed for 15-20 minutes.

In one study, iontophoresis was found to increase the speed of resolution of plantar fasciitis, although it had no effect on long term outcome.

Resting and correcting training errors are critical to the treatment of plantar fasciitis. Patients must modify activities that aggravate this condition; such modifications may be as simple as decreasing the amount, frequency, or intensity of the inciting activity.

Special notes for runners: Runners who overpronate and who have pes planus (flat foot) should select motion-control shoes, which typically feature a more stable construction designed to correct for over-pronation.

Runners who have pes cavus (high arch) should select shoes that have greater cushioning properties.

Extracorporeal shock wave therapy (ESWT) has been proposed as a treatment option for plantar fasciitis. There appears to be few, if any, adverse side effects from this treatment modality. However, to date, results from studies are mixed.

A strengthening program that emphasizes intrinsic foot muscle strengthening is important.

In cases of severe plantar fasciitis, corticosteroid injection may be considered. Other causes of heel pain should also be considered, and a plain x-ray of the foot should always be obtained before injecting steroids.

A corticosteroid injection may be given with ultrasound guidance. Studies have reported success rates of 70 percent or better. Potential risks include plantar fascia rupture and fat pad atrophy. This is the procedure of choice at our center for patients with plantar fasciitis.

The use of platelet-rich plasma (autologous tissue graft) injected into the plantar fascia is thought to stimulate an acute inflammatory reaction that leads to an improvement of the healing process. This treatment has been shown to be effective in a number of limited studies.

Night splints or casts are designed to keep the ankle in a neutral position during sleep. As a result there is passive stretching of the calf and the plantar fascia for a prolonged period.

The night splint allows the plantar fascia to heal in the stretched position, which, in turn, decreases the tension on the fascia with the first step in the morning. A night splint can be molded from either plaster or fiberglass casting material, or a prefabricated and commercially produced plastic brace can be used.

Studies have shown that approximately 80 percent of patients using night splints had improvement of their plantar fasciitis. The splints are especially useful in individuals who have had symptoms of plantar fasciitis for longer than 12 months.

To minimize the chances of reoccurrence of plantar fasciitis, athletes should continue on a maintenance program of daily stretching and/or strengthening at least 2-3 times per week.

Other treatment may include orthotic devices and arch supports.

A relatively new treatment modality involves the use of ultrasound guided tenotomy and, as mentioned above, injection of platelet-rich plasma (autologous tissue grafting). This technique works well.

Patients with low arch place increased stress on the plantar fascia with walking and running. Methods which can avert these problems include taping of the arches, over-the-counter arch supports, and custom orthotic devices. Studies have found significant benefit to these conservative treatments when used in appropriate patients.

For cases that do not respond to conservative treatment, a surgical release of the plantar fascia may be considered. Overall, surgical release has a 70-90 percent success rate in treating patients with this condition; open, endoscopic, or radiofrequency techniques may be used.

Potential complications of surgical intervention include flattening of the longitudinal arch and loss of feeling in the heel.

Other foot tendonitis

The anterior tibial tendon helps control the front of the foot when it meets the ground. If this tendon is strained, a patient may feel pain when they go down stairs or walk or run on hills.

Pain is felt on the top of the foot or at the front of the ankle. There is usually swelling and tenderness on exam.

While the diagnosis may be suspected from the history (sudden increase in athletic activity, etc.), it can be confirmed using diagnostic ultrasound or magnetic resonance imaging. Plain x-rays may be warranted to exclude stress fracture.

Once the diagnosis has been established, the treatment involves the use of rest, ice, anti-inflammatory drugs, and physical therapy.

It is rare that this type of tendonitis becomes very severe.

Special procedures

There are two procedures that many physicians, even specialists, aren't aware of for treating tendonitis. The first is hydrodissection. With this procedure, a large amount of fluid consisting of a mixture of lidocaine, a local anesthetic, glucocorticoid, and sterile saline are used to "peel away" the tendon from the sheath. Oftentimes, tendonitis is due to inflammation of the synovium that lines the tendon sheath and the tendon sticks to the sheath. When it sticks, it causes problems such as trigger finger.

By using hydrodissection, this problem is relieved almost instantly. Hydrodissection must be performed using a small gauge needle and ultrasound guidance by a well-trained physician.

Another procedure that is even more involved is tenotomy. I've mentioned this procedure earlier but I'd like to explain it in more detail. Tenotomy is sometimes done by orthopedic surgeons by opening up the tendon sheath and slicing into the tendon.

But now, it is not necessary to do something so radical. Using a small needle and ultrasound guidance, tenotomy can be performed simply and easily with just local anesthetic.

In addition to doing this, blood is drawn from the patient and spun in a special centrifuge in order to isolate platelet-rich plasma from the blood.

Platelets are blood cells that are rich in a number of growth factors including transforming growth factor beta, fibroblast growth factor, platelet-derived growth factor, epidermal growth factor, vascular endothelial growth factor, and connective tissue growth factor. These growth factors stimulate the synthesis and growth of collagen, an important constituent of tendon tissue.

The platelet-rich plasma is then injected into the tenotomized area after the procedure. Activation of platelets leads to three necessary stages of healing including inflammation, proliferation, and remodeling. There is actual healing of the tendon that takes place.

Conclusion

Tendonitis is an extremely common condition. It represents both a response to overuse as well as a response to degeneration. Over time tendonitis can become chronic. Treatment for tendonitis is dependent on making a proper diagnosis and then treating the condition appropriately.

For more information on tendonitis, contact us at:

Arthritis Treatment Center
71 Thomas Johnson Drive
Frederick, Maryland 21702
(301) 694-5800
(301) 694-0187 Fax
www.arthritistreatmentcenter.com
www.tendonitisandprp.com

You may email me at:
nwei@arthritistreatmentcenter.com

If you want to know more about tendonitis, go to
http://thebookonprp.com/specialoffer/ (password: specialoffer)
for… The Book on PRP.

Here's some of what you'll discover…

- Why poking holes in a tendon is absolutely important to getting results with PRP. Sounds crazy but it's true!
- What medicines should you never ever take before getting PRP!
- How many platelets do you really need to get the result you want? … Discover this number and make sure your doctor swears - this is what you're getting!
- The failsafe, flawless method for delivering PRP… If your doctor isn't using this, run the other way!
- When won't PRP work… you better know the answer to this!

You can get it in print format to read or you can get it as an audio book… or both depending on what you prefer.

The book is not expensive… only $14.99. It's 80 pages long with illustrations. And the audio book – read by me- is $19.99. And if you want to get both it is only $29.99. Plus, take an additional $5.00 off.

Copy the following link on to your internet browser to take advantage of these incredible savings and how PRP therapy may help you!

http://thebookonprp.com/specialoffer/ (password: specialoffer)

www.ingramcontent.com/pod-product-compliance
Lightning Source LLC
Chambersburg PA
CBHW072213280526
45788CB00002B/1002